Be a Superior Life Ace

Step by step instructions to Carry on with A LONG AND Solid LIFE

By

Robert S. Walsh

Be a Superior Life Ace

Would you like to live longer, more joyful, and better? Well assuming this is the case then, at that point, get up out of that seat after you wrap up perusing this report and set those muscles to work. Presently, you can take enhancements or diet pills the entire day, yet without exercise you are just filling your stomach related framework with "hard ball" sprinters that will set aside some margin to process. Without a doubt, certain nature enhancements can help you, yet it takes more than popping pills. Practice is where it is working out, alongside a low-fat, low-fiber diet and a will to reside toward great wellbeing. Obviously, you will likewise have to remove those terrible things to do, for example, smoking, drinking unnecessarily, or utilizing drugs. The medications incorporate over utilization of professionally prescribed drugs. Great wellbeing arrives at those that deal with their sanctuary. (Body) When you work to great wellbeing, thus great wellbeing will come to you in numerous ways. Before you know it,you will find your self doing things you never did.

Contents

Chapter 1:

Step by step instructions to Carry on with A LONG AND Solid LIFE

The future in and all over the planet is expanding every day. Here are far to assist an individual with carrying on with a long solid life. Simply figure how pleasant it is live until you are eighty years of age, or longer.

Practicing good eating habits: Sustenance, nutrients and the right food will assist you with living the age you might want to live. The body needs food to work, and with out a legitimate eating regimen we will be starving indispensable organs from working. Gorging is poor for the body and makes the heart work harder. A few specialists and other wellbeing experts guarantee eating the right food sources that are good for you is more critical than working out.

Practice on a day to day bases will build chances of one getting fragile bones and firm joints when you progress in years. Working out can give your heart a decent speed, which assists you with proceeding with a better way of life without feeling drowsy. Stress and uneasiness can diminished with work out.

3

 On the off chance that you are not doing any activity at the present time, begin now. Try not to get into enormous exercises to begin with. Doing basic arm lifts, leg lifts, even extending. Go all over steps in the event that you can utilize steps at a sluggish speed two or multiple times. Following seven days you can acquaint your body with somewhat more work out. Take as much time as is needed.

Dozing will assist with body capabilities, less pressure, and tension. Rest assists you with thinking obviously. Get a decent daily schedule for resting. Figure out how much rest you truly need. During the day, maybe you on the off chance that are not working, you could lay down for a brief rest, which could assist you with feeling significantly improved during the night. Everybody is unique so you should find out for yourself your body's expectation's for rest.

Drink a lot of water. Water will assist with completing poisons, other related bugs and things that your framework needn't bother with. Water is the main liquid that will truly flush ones framework out. It is prescribed to hydrate ordinary. Recollect whenever you are out and require something to drink. Pause and get a container of water. You will set aside cash and your wellbeing with out sugar, carbon and different fixings in a pop.

Safeguard your self from risks that can hurt you. Do you get a kick out of the chance to ride a bicycle? Do you wear a protective cap? Try not to say goodness that is not really for me. Today the two youngsters and grown-ups are harmed regularly with bicycle mishaps. Safeguard your head and why not your mind.

Stress, despondency, and nervousness: These are things that an individual ought to truly chip away at and contemplate to lessen pressure, discouragement and uneasiness in their life. Besides the fact that it hurting is you, it is making pressure the heart. We want to figure out how to live with these things and figure out how to unwind.

Smoking you should surrender it. Not much to say regarding that. It isn't great, smells awful, and tastes terrible. Your heart and lungs could do without it. Surrender it.

Keep the physical check-ups. See your PCP as frequently as they would like you to go. Have yearly check ups to guarantee that things are good with you. We want to adopt a strategy of preventive consideration.

Utilize great creams and moisturizers to safeguard the skin from a lot of sun. Creams and lotions will assist with keeping solid skin. As we age the skin will begin to separate and disperse.

With utilizing a decent salve and creams on you skin the entire body will assist with keeping your skin in the right equilibrium. Become familiar with how to live longer and better.

Chapter 2 :

<u>**Step by step instructions to Carry on with A More drawn out AND More joyful LIFE**</u>

Numerous scholars spread data across the channels of the Web letting you know how they feel you can live longer, better and more joyful. The truth of the matter is assuming that you need joy you need to reach inside and pull up your normal assets and permit them to direct you to joy.

In any case, in the event that you need to live longer and better you should adjust to another way of life, which is liberated from drugs, synthetics, substances, specific propensities and direct, etc. You should exercise to increase digestion, bones, joints, and muscles.

As people we really want profound food, mental, and actual food sources to keep us better areas of strength for and. Otherworldly food incorporates supplication, a more profound significance of the insights from God, and progressing tidiness of the brain and body.

6

 The body is our sanctuary and in the event that we eat or drink unsafe medications or unnecessary liquor, as well as take part in destructive activities we will endure wretchedness, chronic frailty, and our life expectancy will abbreviate.

Living longer, better and cheerful requires exertion. At the point when you apply self to living longer, better and more joyful likely you will accomplish. In any case, you want objectives, plans, and activity to find the ways to push toward great wellbeing.

We can examine many subtleties to assist you with figuring out how to live longer, more joyful, and better. A portion of the things we do in life can really hurt us. In the event that we don't accomplish appropriate rest it can extra time cause heart issues, as well as other ailments.

The beginning of each and every wellbeing plan is eating right and getting legitimate rest. At the point when you digest quality food sources with the legitimate nutrients and enhancements you can develop to a better life. The issue is these days FDA is permitting unhealthier fixings in our food that it is influencing millions.

One reason that weight is expanding is because of specialists added to meats, which cause desires.

7

 To assist you with nutrients we can consider a couple of subtleties, still you really want to consider halting and beginning new wellbeing examples to push toward better living.

A couple of different things we can consider is understanding personalities, practicing, judging, separating, exhort, fantasizes, mollifies, fighting, crashes, being correct, etc. A great many people neglect to see that the manner in which they act could cause pressure, which makes them troubled.

Many individuals stay away from earnestness. At the point when a discussion becomes serious an individual could wreck by ignoring the data, or, more than likely kidding. While you might think this is a method for lessening pressure, the truth of the matter is crashing just sets an individual up for some tumbles to come.

Some of the time you must be serious and it checks out. While you might need to get away from the real world, the truth of the matter is one day you will wake and smell the no-nonsense realities of the real world, and when it smacks you in the face so hard, you will think back and wish you hadn't gone through your time on earth wrecking.

Once more, many individuals stand by listening to what they need to hear and overlook what they wish to keep away from.

8

At the point when this happens we have a sifting framework, which bit by bit you will carry on with an existence of wretchedness, essentially on the grounds that when your boat rolls in you will be out in the sea swimming without gear.

At times we need to acknowledge the obvious issues. On the off chance that you are drinking exorbitantly and your companions or family fills you in about, pay attention to what they are talking about, since you are not just harming you, you are harming your loved ones.

Generally, we really want profound, supplements, nutrients, work out, and legitimate ways of behaving to carry on with a solid, longer, and more joyful way of life.

Chapter 3:
Instructions to LIVE HAPPIERHOW TO LIVE LONGER, Better AND More joyful

Did you had at least some idea that profound reactions can send pessimistic reaction, which can make an individual troubled? When an individual is miserable, did you had any idea that it lessens life length, as well as wellbeing?

One of the ways of working on your life and live better is to figure out how to effectively tune in. At the point when you figure out how to listen effectively you lessen sifting, crashing, fantasizing, assuaging, etc. Keeping away from these propensities will build your reasoning, as well as assist you with perceiving how you can live longer, better and more joyful.

Different ways can assist you with living more joyful, including figuring out how to summarize while speaking with others. Frequently connections go to pieces while inert listening happens. For example, when a lady is disturbed you might strike out sincerely at her mate, which he answers with negative returns. This all prompts misery, and will cause medical issues, which your life will abbreviate.

At the point when you rework during correspondence you sum up the thing is being said. At the point when you rehash data frequently it explains correspondence, which creates a much useful relationship. We can see a couple of tests to assist you with perceiving how summarizing can lessen contention.

Rework:

Sarah: Joe, I needed to purchase another dress for the impending occasion.

Joe: You need another dress?

Sarah: All things considered, indeed, I would like another dress.

Joe: In this way, you are saying you need to buy another dress for the impending occasion. (Explaining), in this way, you are inquiring as to whether purchasing the dress is alright.

Sarah: Yes dear,

Joe: I'm fine with that, in the event that you need another dress get one. Sarah: Much obliged.

This is a straightforward reword, yet you can perceive how it eliminates any confusion. Summarizing will stop dormant tuning in. Summarizing will likewise address any claims, presumptions, or misread correspondence. At the point when you reword you additionally make each other cheerful, since you will feel appreciated and recognized.

11

Correspondence works the two different ways, and on the off chance that you reword you can lessen irate feelings, which frequently raise when data is misconstrued. Rewording is an effective method for expanding memory too.

At what time feelings commotion, it influences the heart, which frequently prompts chronic frailty. Assuming you need to live longer, better, and more joyful, you need to get a handle on feelings. Explaining is one more method for controlling feelings, which advances better living. At the point when you figure out how to reword, it will take you to explanation.

While pursuing summarizing and explaining you need to ensure you have unadulterated expectations. At the point when you explain, or state you need to abstain from accusing, controlling, and criticism (disparaging) your accomplice, or who you speak with.

Negative energy will just prompt medical conditions, breakdown in connections, etc. Negative energy is awful, which prompts despondency, deter, outrage, and skeptical reasoning. Fundamentally, pessimistic feelings are disavowal and refusal in synopsis. In truth, pessimistic energy is an enormous issue that is making individuals endure.

12

A portion of the outcomes from pessimistic energy (profound reaction) are cardiovascular breakdown, hypertension, strokes, coronary failures, etc. As you can see figuring out how to utilize undivided attention strategies can assist you with living longer, better, and more joyful.

It's valid. At the point when you figure out how to foster good energy you will sparkle like a star, which will encourage you inside. To develop to shrewd reasoning, (Utilizing the psyche to think, as opposed to the feelings) you can likewise figure out how to work on paying attention to criticism. At the point when you give or get input you won't utilize judgment, negative analysis, etc. Rather, you will have unadulterated expectations while tuning in or giving criticism. As you figure out how to summarize you will construct abilities, for example, explaining and criticism. Living longer, better and more joyful is turning into an overall interest these days.

Chapter 4 :

Instructions to LIVE More joyful, LONGER AND Better Self improvement Devices

We can examine work out, sustenance, nutrients, etc, and we can move to live better, more joyful, and longer. In any case, we really want to think about propensities, ways of behaving, thinking, and direct to carry on with a more full way of life.

A few ways of behaving many individuals adjust to incorporate pacifying, fighting, in every case right, fantasizes, crashing, channels, understanding personalities, guidance, practicing, judging, etc.

In the word we have battles, contentions, and separations in homes, as well as harassing and conflicts in school. The issue is breakdowns in correspondence, disavowal, and improper ways of behaving, propensities, thinking, activities, etc. In some cases when couples are together for a time span they will frequently make dreams or dream, in this manner floating away from their accomplice.

This frequently prompts breakdown in connections, and it is an uncalled for, low demonstration against someone else. Sure we as a whole fantasy or jump out briefly, yet when we take it excessively far and use it as an endeavor to get away from the real world, we are just hurting. In the event that you need to live longer, better and more joyful you should change this type of conduct as well as propensity.

One of the normal issues we face today is individuals neglecting to hear a whole story, or, in all likelihood removing individuals before have the opportunity to complete the process of talking. Frequently individuals miss the in the middle of between the correspondence. For example, John unexpectedly cut Sherri off when she was enlightening him concerning her work over-burden.

John would have rather not caught wind of issues, so he immediately moved the discussion to what he did that day. This is discourteous when all Sherri required was a touch of solace and conceivable agree to permit her feelings and sentiments to show.

15

Mollifying works similarly, for example frequently messages in correspondence is missed. At the point when an individual pacifies they work to lessen outrage, by making statements that satisfies the individual.

Quite possibly of the biggest issue on the planet is judging. Scores of individuals judge and seldom do they genuinely get to know the individual they judge. For example, a neighbourhood young lady, for quite a long time was denounced, called indecent names, and around a decade not too far off individuals watched her ways of behaving and profoundly apologized. While harming was finished, not one individual more than decade had sufficient sense to quit judging. Making a decision about makes the feelings ruckus, which prompts uncertainty, dread, and pessimistic energy. To carry on with a more drawn out, better, and more joyful life, quit passing judgment on others.

Many individuals read minds. That is they frequently put words in the mouth of others, as opposed to hearing what is really shared with them. For example, Jerry let Lisa know that her hair looked great. Lisa quietly thought, "He could do without the manner in which I did my hair today." When somebody says your hair looks great, how could you believe that the individual is lying? At the point when you want to guess what people groups might be thinking, you might need to find a new line of work and go On the planet's Book of Family.

16

As you can see ways of behaving, thinking designs, propensities, direct, and such requirements acclimating to carry on with a more drawn out, better, and more joyful life. At the point when you permit such ways of behaving to control your brain, what you are doing is cursing your wellbeing.

In any case, you should work out, eat right, and stop different propensities that could prompt chronic weakness. For example, in the event that you drink unreasonably or neglect to practice your wellbeing will steadily break down which in time you will feel hopeless. Exercise to live longer and better.

Chapter 5 :

Step by step instructions to LIVE Better AND LONGER HOW TO LIVE More joyful

We as a whole go through days when the world appears to tumble on our shoulders. As of now we might feel living better, longer, and more joyful is far off. A few of us manage pressure as it comes our direction, while others find it hard to deal with. The issue lies with what? Stress is a day to day factor that we as a whole should confront every day. There is no chance to get out of pressure. Assuming you figure out how to limit stressors and lessen pressure it can assist you with living longer, better, and more joyful. One of the most mind-blowing ways of decreasing pressure is performing stretch activities. In light of this we can get familiar with a couple of supportive tips to train you a couple of stretch activities to decrease pressure. At the point when you practice customary activity, you are attempting to help energy, rest sounder, support confidence, etc.

Stress minimizers

Pose: The stance is significant. At the point when the stance is in great working condition you can frequently sit no less than ten minutes without feeling uncomfortable.

Before you start practice you ought to constantly check your stance, which ought to be adjusted.

Relaxing:

Stretch activities and contemplation require appropriate relaxing. While getting ready to live longer, better, and more joyful you need to inhale normally while playing out any activity, contemplation, etc.

<u>***Meditation***</u>:

Before starting exercise you may want to practice meditation. Meditation helps to clear your mind and enforce positive thinking. You will need to practice focusing your attention while performing meditation practices. Some people prefer to listen to easy sounds, while others focus better on objects. You will want to make a choice before practicing meditation.

<u>***Attitude***</u>:

Your attitude plays a part in living healthier, longer, and happier. When you have a positive outlook or attitude it moves you to achieve your goals and plans to live longer, healthier, and happier. To start meditation and stretches sit in the floor.

19

We can start with the Lotus Position, i.e. unless you have an injured back. You can still perform the meditation practice, yet you may have to sit in a different fashion. While performing the Lotus meditation practice, sit on the floor. Make sure the posture is straight. Now with open palms place your hands upright on your knees, while you lock your legs. When you first sit in the floor, make sure your legs are stretched to the front. Next, you want to bend the knee and use your hand to grasp your right foot. You want to bring the foot in toward the abdominal, by placing it upon your thigh. (Left)

Perform the same action on the right foot. (Buddha Meditation) The Lotus Position Meditation is a Buddha practice. During the process you want to, once the feet are in place, you want to make sure the knees are touching the floor, while the feet scales turn upward. Make sure posture and head is in alignment.

Relax the stomach muscles. While the palms are turned upward and resting on your knees, touch the thumbs on each finger, joining them with the pointing finger. Now you can start meditation. If you lit a candle to focus on, thus focus on the object and allow the mind to freely let go of thoughts.

20

<u>**NOTE**</u>: You may want to stretch a couple of times before performing Lotus Position Meditation. This will help the muscles flex with ease.

Practicing meditation will boost your awareness, as well as promote relaxation. When the mind and body relaxes, it promotes health, life span, and happiness. If you are uncomfortable with this type of Lotus Meditation, you may want to consider the Half Lotus, or the Perfect Posture positions. Mediation is a surefire way to help you live longer, happier, and healthier.

chapter 6 :

HOW TO LIVE LONGER AND HEALTHIER WITH EXERCISE

If you want to live longer and healthier you will need to put forth effort that will make you feel better. You cannot live a lifestyle of drinking, smoking and all those other nasty words and expect to live longer and healthier life.

One of the best things you can do to live longer is to exercise and eat right. The problem is nowadays the FDA is putting harmful stuff in our foods that is causing fatalities and few are recognizing what is truly going on. Diabetes is one of the leading health problems causing death, yet cures are available, the FDA and Pharmacists are fighting it because they prefer to make money, rather than save lives.

Recently, I learnt that if you adhere to a fiber-based food you can beat diabetes, or else minimize the symptoms of diabetes. Now, most people are not going to tell you this because, (we won't speak names) but they would prefer you to rely on prescriptions or drugs to survive an illness. The fact is you can use natural substances to survive.

22

Still, the only problem is sprays and other harmful chemicals are contaminating nature.

What are we to do? We have the choice, and that is to exercise and do our best to eat the foods that will not contaminate our bodies. We have to fight in other words to live longer and healthier, simply because the truth is, man is causing his own injury. We can grow our own vegetables and fruits, which we can avoid harmful chemicals that will pollute such natural vitamins. Still, we need to work the muscles, bones, joints, and other elements of our body to survive what man is destroying. Exercise is proven to enhance health and life. Exercise helps us to grow stronger and live healthier. To understand this we must understand how the body functions. We must understand that joints, bones, muscles, cells, blood, and all that good stuff plays a large part in how we can live longer and healthier.

The body has ways that tell us what we need. When the body does not receive what it needs it will let us know. When the body tells us what it needs and we neglect to do anything about it, guess what? We experience suffering. We experience illness.

23

We experience pain, and eventually we end up on medications that help to determine which direction our lives will go. The body has metabolism, pineal glands, blood, cells, tissues, joints, and more. While you may think that the muscles and bones is essential to protect, the fact you need to protect the joints first, since the joints affect the bones and muscles and if you injure a cartilage (joint) you would have done damage to the bones and muscles. When you injure the muscles and bones, you have problems. Still, the spine (Central Nervous System) is affected; we have ongoing illness, which deteriorates the life. WE have a problem. Now if you want to live longer and healthier, you will need to protect the CNS-Central Nervous System, otherwise you are in serious trouble.

This is where exercise comes in. If you perform proper exercise you 46an protect and strengthening the spine, and in turn you will build life and health. You may eat the foods contaminated, yet when you exercise you open up airways that will not open with foods and in turn, you have a security that will walk the dog. You build resistance, strength, and metabolism. This is what you want to focus on while considering living longer and healthier in life. Reducing stress can help you live longer, healthier, and happier.

Chapter 7 :

A DIRECTIVE FOR HEALTHIER LIVING: HOW TO DECREASE STRESS TO LIVE LONGER AND HAPPIER

You can live longer, healthier, and happier if you reduce your stress. Happiness frequently follows desire of a longer, healthier life. Stress is pressure, or a physiological reaction, to which the body and mind will react when pressure arises. When stress arises, a person typically feels challenged, threatened, or afraid of change. We must work twice as hard to survive nowadays, which has increased the prevalence of ailments brought on by stress. Today's pain affects considerably more people than 1 million people annually.

However, stress can have a positive impact. When under stress, try to shift your thoughts from being negative to being optimistic. how it functions

First, always remind yourself that you are sufficient because no one can predict what tomorrow will bring. Additionally, until you are completely stressed out, practice living one day at a time. Then, practice living one second at a time.

Consider utilizing healthier coping mechanisms if you frequently turn to alcohol or drugs to ease anxiety. If you are having trouble sleeping and find that alcohol puts you to sleep, keep in mind that drinking causes you to lose REM sleep. The crucial dream state occurs during REM.

You can buy melatonin supplements at your neighbourhood pharmacy, which will calm your tensions and aid in falling asleep. The few dollars you spend on melatonin will be more than offset by the money you'll save not using alcohol or drugs to unwind. We can go through a few specifics now if you are not familiar with stress indicators, emotional symptoms, mental symptoms, physical symptoms, or stress-related behaviours.

The Symptoms

An excessive amount of stress can make a person irritable. It's likely that you are stressed out when you feel tense, anxious, or impatient. Stress symptoms include sensitivity, gloomy thinking, and taking offense at what others say to you. You may be under stress if you are fidgeting, biting your nails, pulling your hair, or jiggling your knees. Stress-related symptoms include nausea, diarrhoea, constipation, and frequent smoking.

26

Insomniac Symptoms

When you frequently forget things or have trouble focusing, your mind is probably overloaded with thoughts. Similar to this, if you have trouble making decisions of any kind and find yourself obsessing, you're probably under a lot of stress. Stress manifests as exhaustion and intense pressure feelings.

Mood Disorders:

Low self-esteem, anxiety, panic attacks, wrath, resentment, being ready to cry frequently, moodiness, nightmares, and an inability to laugh are a few examples of emotional symptoms associated with stress.

Physical symptoms or physiology:

Muscle tightness and weariness may be present while you're under stress. Back, head, shoulder, and neck aches are likely to occur. Your eyelids could feel heavy and the muscles in the corners of your eyes might spasm. Frequently, the mouth feels dry and the jaw feels rigid. The fingers frequently feel cold whereas the palms of the hands frequently feel sweaty. You can frequently have stomach, bladder, and urine issues, as well as heartburn.

27

When you are under a lot of stress, you could also have heart palpitations, weight gain or loss, headaches, colds, hyperventilation, and other symptoms.

behavioural indicators

When under extreme stress, people frequently become enraged and violent when miscommunications take place. The individual may speak aggressively, with frequent interruptions of other people. The person may occasionally withdraw from social situations or groups. The individual can quit taking care of themselves and display obsessive-compulsive traits.

As you can see, stress poses a risk to your health, happiness, and quality of life unless you learn to harness it for positive effects.

Chapter 8:

<u>BE HEALTHY AND LIVE A LONGER LIFE</u>

Human life is in danger from aging. It undermines our advantages and deprives us of life's pleasures. The devastating effects of aging finally result in our deaths. Each year, millions of people who have age-related health problems pass away.

Fewer individuals are aware that diet and lifestyle changes can reasonably reduce degenerative aging, just as they can do for many medical diseases. Few people are aware of the scientific research being done on this ailment, which aims to one day intervene in the aging process to treat the condition.

29

A healthy life increase is what? You may live longer if you use research to lengthen a healthier lifetime and learn to reduce the hazards of worrying about getting older-related problems. Utilizing the most effective methods available now while encouraging research to produce methods that are more efficient in the future.

For their patients to have a healthier and longer life, doctors and scientists encourage a balanced diet, conforming lifestyles, diverse technological tactics, and novel medical discoveries. When you stop to think about it, there is more to a healthy life span than simply eating the appropriate foods and exercising regularly.

The treatments available now fall well short of what is required by researchers. Finding funding for research will aid in the future development of medications by helping to educate the public.

Living a long life gives you more time to keep fit and alive. The public will be able to receive a better education and live longer, healthier lives because to scientific research and capacity.

30

What can I do to prolong my life?

Healthy eating, frequent exercise, following your doctor's recommendations for regular checkups, and perhaps a change in lifestyle would be beneficial.

Are you a smoker? Stop doing this since it increases your risk of developing lung ailments, cancer, blood vessel occlusion, and other conditions.

31

Are you an alcoholic? Do you regularly consume alcohol? Alcohol consumption will damage your liver, make you depressed, and prematurely age your skin and outer look.

Do you use illicit substances? Using illegal substances initially is prohibited. Secondhand illegal narcotics create stress and strain on key organs, causing them to not operate properly. Once you quit using drugs illegally and get older, some side effects may appear. Vital organs will be impacted, the brain may not function as well, your vision may be compromised, or the heart may no longer be able to withstand the usage of drugs you used to abuse when you were younger.

Do you often use over-the-counter medications, prescription medications that a friend or your doctor may have given you, or both, and feel that the dosage is insufficient? You will die from this. Most people are unaware that excessive drug usage may stress, strain, and cause essential organs to work harder or slower, can contaminate the blood stream, and result in improper brain function. To treat a specific sickness or condition, medications are prescribed. A medication can have serious negative effects for anyone if the side effects and actual nature are not known.

32

Not everyone can take all sorts of medications because they are allergic to certain of them, and some people cannot take medications because of specific medical conditions.

A person can get started on the proper path to promoting themselves to a longer and healthier life by taking a look at some of these questions. Your chances of living a happier and longer life will increase if you give up any or all of your bad habits.

You can start right now by doing some study to find out more about your habits. Find out for yourself what could happen and the implications of prolonged use. Make an appointment with your doctor immediately away by giving them a call. Inform them of your habit or addiction. Your doctor can assist you in finding the correct resources and set you up for a happier, healthier, longer life.

Change your life today. You'll be happy you did.

Chapter 9:

HOW TO RELATE TO STRESS WILL HELP YOU LIVE LONGER AND HEALTHIER

The leading stressor that can benefit everyone is emotional stress.

A person may suffer several kinds of stress, including mental stress, bodily stress, and emotional stress. The body and mind might suffer negative side effects from excessive stress. A life without stress can be boring as well. One can see the issues or circumstances with a person who may be feeling stressed or nervous by taking a look at a normal week. Finding the issue or circumstance will enable someone to deal with it and resolve it.

Do you worry for a half-hour every day? This might be a positive encounter. According to doctors, worrying for 30 minutes a day can help you feel less worried. Do you worry a lot? You won't have to worry anymore because people who worry a lot don't usually have more serious problems than others. We only believe that we are dealing with more serious issues and attempt to manage them without giving them any thought.

Exercise frequently and intensify your efforts. Why? Exercise will help give lifelong expectancy with the aging process by slowing it down. When a person looks and feels wonderful, they will feel less stress and have more confidence. Daily exercise will keep you healthier and help you feel less stressed.

If you don't move your joints and muscles, arthritis will develop. The body and lengthy life span may suffer as a result. As a person ages, their joints will tighten up, their muscles will weaken, and their external look will change. By exercising, a person can maintain their joints flexible and prevent fragile bones from breaking from falls as they age. As the majority of us are aware, hips may break extremely easily with even a small fall as we age.

Reading a good book can teach you how to relax, which is believed to help reduce stress. Your mind will be distracted from daily worries by reading. causing the body to unwind by stretching its muscles and allowing its limp joints to do nothing. listening to music, perhaps just the sound of water falling, a storm, or your favourite CD. Put your eyes closed and unwind. Perhaps all you need is a decent crossword puzzle or a relaxing activity to help you decompress after a long day. One benefit of relaxing is that it will make life's obstacles easier to handle.

35

Do you have a hard time falling asleep? Are you getting adequate rest? Sleeping is essential for lowering daily stress. Getting a new mattress may help you get the rest you need because mattresses may contribute to sleep deprivation. Even your bedroom, including the comforter, sheets, and other furnishings, may be changed. Making restful sleeping a habit might help you feel less stressed and live a longer, healthier life.

Eating well: Eating well will enhance a person's quality of life in every manner. Eating is essential for maintaining a healthy, functional body by providing it with the necessary vitamins, iron, lipids, and carbohydrates. A body can become sluggish without the right foods and nutrients; organs can suffer damage without the right foods; and the brain can not work well without food.

Healthy living includes eating the right foods for your body, getting enough sleep, learning how to relax, and exercising to prevent stiffness and arthritis in your joints. As a person ages, all of these wonderful features will help them cope with stress, live long and happy lives, and stay healthy, free from high blood pressure, high cholesterol, and other heart-related diseases. It is not too late to start with a healthy life to expand your life with aging.

36

Check with your doctor for more information; do research on the internet for more tips and ideas with staying healthy. HGH (Human Growth Hormone) can also help you live longer, healthier, and happier.

Chapter 10 :

HGH PRODUCTS CAN HELP YOU LIVE LONGER, HEALTHIER, AND HAPPIER

I recently conducted in-depth research on HGH (Human Growth Hormone), and as I looked into the specifics of this hormone, I learned that having a balanced level of HGH can help you live longer, healthier lives.

Human growth hormone (HGH), which is created by the body's endocrine glands, controls the chemicals that are present in us. Alternately, the substance targets specific cells, stimulating or regulating them to increase metabolism. (Force that Sustains Life) Growth and development are supported by the regulation of our bodies by human growth hormones. The hormones maintain our youth. The hormones that are released by our pituitary glands then pass through the liver and transform into the anti-aging hormone IGF-1 (Insulin Growth Factor). Since hormones control the body's glucose level, insulin is crucial.

Insulin secretes through "islets of langerhans" into the pancreas, which regulates glucose. When glucose is deficient it can result into diabetes or diabetes mellitus.

DHEA is then produced by the pineal glands. Every ten years, the body's hormone synthesis mechanism begins to slow down (DEHYDROEPIANDROSTERONE). Therefore, you might want to think about HGH pills in addition to supplements that contain DHEA if you want to live longer, better, and happier. Melatonin is a hormone that is secreted by the pineal glands and has an impact on the bloodstream and brain.

We can take supplements as well as a healthy diet to increase our hormone levels. Diet and supplements will be enhanced by appropriate activity. You must therefore exert effort if you want to live longer, be healthier, and be happier. Setting up a program for exercise, food, and supplements can be challenging for most people, but once you get going, it gets simpler with each step toward a longer, healthier, and happier life.

One of the best things about HGH is that it will aid in weight loss and improve muscular tone. Additionally, the vitamins will help you increase your power, stamina, and energy levels, which is fantastic for extending your life and improving your health. Happiness comes with a longer, healthier life.

39

You can reduce aging symptoms, such as wrinkles, by exercising, eating healthfully, and taking supplements like HGH. Above all, you will get restorative sleep, which is an advantage that will lengthen your life and make it healthier and happier. Additionally, taking supplements will help you reduce cholesterol, strengthen your heart, increase bone density, and enhance your brain's functions.

Supplements, nutrition, exercise, and other factors are important, but we also need to think about unhealthy habits and behaviors that can shorten our lives. For instance, if you overeat, drink excessively, use drugs, stay up late, and so on, you are shortening your life expectancy. You must choose a lifestyle that frees you from unhealthy living if you want to live longer, better, and happier lives.

As soon as you begin to live a healthy lifestyle, you will notice an improvement in your mood. You will get stronger with every step you take, which will help you live longer and be healthier. Additionally, since stressors cause stress, you should attempt to decrease them. You can achieve this by changing your emotions and focusing on positive energies with your thoughts rather than dwelling on negative ones. Negative energy just shorten life.

40

You can live longer, healthier, and happier if you work to change your mindset and incorporate supplements into your diet and workout routine.

Visit the Internet where a wealth of knowledge is waiting for you to discover more about HGH, different workout regimens, diets, supplements, and other topics. To find out what diet and exercise are best for you, you should also talk to your doctor. You can attain success by learning how to live longer, healthier, and happier.

41

Tips for Living a Longer and Healthier Life How to Live a Longer and Healthier Life

Age becomes our enemy as we become older. We lose strength as we age because our muscles and joints become weaker. Aging robs us of the pleasures we formerly experienced in life while also slowing down our metabolism. Aging finally becomes a crippler that saps our bodies of their life energy. Millions of individuals pass away from old age every year, and the ageing population is growing at an accelerating rate.

Degenerative aging is the process of getting older, but recent research suggests that we can halt it. By maintaining a healthy diet, making lifestyle and habit changes, and following medical recommendations that will help us live longer, healthier lives, we can control or at least slow down the aging process. Recent studies are demonstrating scientific practices that have been shown to slow aging. The researchers are making great efforts to comprehend aging while employing aging intervention strategies. New discoveries should result in happier, healthier, and longer lives.

42

The process of scientific measures nowadays results in a healthy life extension, where the formulae discovered greatly expand life span as the actions taken lower the hazards of age-related pain. Science is now putting great effort into finding ways to make people live longer, better lives while also delaying aging because the conditions frequently result in serious health issues and ultimately death.

 In order to delay aging, news media, health spas, physicians, and others are encouraging food, exercise, healthier lifestyles, and doing so while utilizing cutting-edge technological methods and medical breakthroughs.

How we can help:
By keeping informed, we can contribute to the development of innovative anti-aging treatments. We can help support research as well as educate the local populations. The money will assist researchers in creating drugs for future use. A longer lifespan will increase the amount of time we spend learning new things and living healthier lives as we gain more knowledge.

What can I personally do to prolong my life?
Consume a balanced diet, move your body, visit your doctor frequently, and ask for guidance.

43

 To live longer, healthier, and happier, you must also learn to listen and act. We can talk about habits as well.

 Drug, alcohol, and cigarette usage are all unhealthy habits that increase the risk of disease and death. Smoking increases your risk of developing cancer, lung disease, clogged blood vessels, strokes, and other conditions. Drinking too much puts your liver at risk. You may suffer depression, which causes additional problems that will advance aging.

 Using illegal drugs or overtaking prescriptions can cause the vital signs, as well as the organs to function improperly. Stress increases, which often strain the vital organs. Sometimes the affects of smoking, alcohol, and drugs will not show until you advance in age. The vital organs, brain, sight, heart, all in time however will show evidence of your poor living conditions at a youthful age.

 Over-the-counter drugs or prescription drugs is sometimes used as a sedative, or else a "high," which also causes harm. AS you continue to misuse prescription drugs, your vital organs, metabolism, heart, and overall health will diminish. If you are confused about the usage of drugs, prescriptions, alcohol, tobacco, and so forth we encourage you to research to learn more now.

44

Learning is growing, which can help you move to live longer, healthier, and happier. Stopping your bad habits now is a way to grow, live, and stop aging and poor health. You can stop now and move to exercise and diet to live longer, healthier, and happier.

To learn more about living healthier, happier, and longer, continue researching the market and ask your doctor for advice that can help you grow.

Solid SKIN IN HOW TO LIVE LONGER AND More joyful LIVING Better

Did you had any idea that dealing with the skin can assist you with feeling more youthful? At the point when you deal with your skin it assists you with looking better, which advances joy. All things considered, you really want more to carry on with a more extended, better, and more joyful life.

We can examine skin health management, and proposition you a couple of supportive tips to work on your skin to look more youthful, yet you will require work out, diet, a lot of water, and potential enhancements to live longer, better, and more joyful.

Why skin bites the dust:

Maturing is one of the great reasons that the skin starts to bite the dust. However, in the event that you drink low volumes of water, the skin won't have the regular components it requirements to decrease maturing side effects. The skin likewise needs oils, creams, nutrients, and minerals to remain sound. As we become older the epidermis starts to thin and becomes delicate.

Our organs that produce oil decline in discharge, as well as the veins. Old cells are seldom re-established as you become older too, which additionally expands side effects of maturing.

After you figure hereditary qualities, sun contact, synthetics, unfortunate ways of life, exorbitant sun tanning, etc. you will see the reason why individuals look more seasoned than they genuinely are.

Tip:

While saturating the throat region generally apply the moisturizers while utilizing firm, and strokes that move up. Continuously cover the neck and face with sunscreens that incorporate SPF factors, particularly assuming you visit the sun frequently. In the event that you wear low-neck pullovers frequently, women safeguard your chest region with sunscreens also.

Answer:

Dive more deeply into the sorts of pads that can slow wrinkling around the jaw, and neck region.

Tip:

Mayonnaise and Egg Whites and Burdens can fix the skin. To blend mix until the recipe is smooth.

45

The Adversaries:

Sun is the skin's adversary. Be content with what variety God gave you as opposed to over heat in the sun. This will assist you with cleaning seem energetic long into the future. In any case, some sun is solid, since it gives regular proteins that improve the tissue. Sun radiation, as well as other hurtful fixings integrated into the sun will make the skin lose collagen, as well as elastin.

Tip:

Sunscreen is encouraged to lessen wrinkling caused from sun. Sunscreen preliminaries, which incorporate SPF, can likewise assist with limiting kinks, crow feet, and almost negligible differences. The expansive range equations work best.

Answer:

Wearing lip ointments and lipsticks can help battle wrinkling of the lips, which comes from extreme contact of the sun.

Tip:

Wearing a cap when the sun is a lot of can help battle wrinkling, skin malignant growth, etc.

Presently we can think about way of life. On the off chance that you smoke it can make you age quicker, as well as influence your wellbeing.

46

Assuming you need to live longer, better, and more joyful, quit smoking at this point. Support gatherings, spellbinding, and different cures are accessible at the neighbourhood drug store to help you very smoking.

Rest is significant. A great many individuals are doing combating rest problems. Assuming you are battling, engaging a sleeping disorder, rest apnea, or different sorts of rest issues look for help now. You can utilize regular cures, for example, Melatonin to lessen pressure and lay down easily. Different equations or enhancements are accessible to assist you with dozing too. Attempt to remain in the regular cure isle while attempting to live longer, better, and more joyful. Gravity resisting activities can assist you with living longer and better too.

47

GRAVITY Opposing IN HOW TO LIVE LONGER AND Better LIVING More joyful

Weightlifting is a gravity opposing power that assists us with living longer, better, and more joyful. A bunch of hand weights could do marvels to the body. Weightlifting will assist you with diminishing lists, while conditioning, managing, and firming the body.

As we become older the muscles go to fat. At what time the muscles go to fat, the weight frequently causes joint harm. Digestion additionally diminishes as we become older, which decreases our life-supporting power.